Why Your Hair Is

Thinning and How

to Grow It Back

WIGS
SCARVES
&LIES

Myrna J. Buckles

NEW YORK

LONDON • NASHVILLE • MELBOURNE • VANCOUVER

Wigs, Scarves, & Lies
© 2019 Myrna J. Buckles

Published in New York, New York, by Morgan James Publishing in partnership with Difference Press. Morgan James is a trademark of Morgan James, LLC. www.MorganJamesPublishing.com

The Morgan James Speakers Group can bring authors to your live event. For more information or to book an event visit The Morgan James Speakers Group at www.TheMorganJamesSpeakersGroup.com.

ISBN 978-1-64279-032-0 paperback
ISBN 978-1-64279-033-7 eBook
Library of Congress Control Number: 2018941778

Cover & Interior Design by:
Megan Whitney Dillon
Creative Ninja Designs
megan@creativeninjadesigns.com

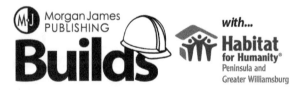

In an effort to support local communities, raise awareness and funds, Morgan James Publishing donates a percentage of all book sales for the life of each book to Habitat for Humanity Peninsula and Greater Williamsburg.

Get involved today! Visit
www.MorganJamesBuilds.com

For Dan, my support and my rock,
even when the path was not clear.

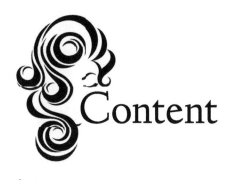

Content

Introduction

"There is no greater thing you can do with your life and your work than follow your passions—in a way that serves the world and you."

SIR RICHARD BRANSON

I know you woke up very early this morning, hours before anyone else in your family even thought about waking up. Every morning you have a routine that includes painstaking attention to every detail of your hair. The fear of being found out drives you. So, you wake up at 4 or 5 am every day, shower, and apply your foundation, mascara, blush, and a little eyeliner so you feel a little more like you used to before you started losing hair. Then you spend the next hour and a half carefully and strategically drying and arranging your hair.

You see yourself in the mirror, and the reflection looking back at you says it's time to get to work disguising your hair loss. You've checked the weather forecast to make sure it isn't going to be overly windy and looked at your schedule multiple times to make sure you haven't overlooked an outside event or activity. Your son has soccer practice tonight, so you know you absolutely can't forget to take the ball cap that goes best with the outfit you chose for today. So many things to think about every single morning, it's draining.

You have a rhythm when you comb your hair in the morning: comb, scoop, comb, scoop, hair into the toilet; comb, scoop, comb, scoop, hair into the toilet. You maximize every strand of your hair as you fix it, this hair over that hair; first you brush left, and then you brush right. Horrified, you notice your part is much wider than you thought, so you move your part one millimeter to the left of where you typically part it. Oops, that won't work, too thin there, so you go a millimeter to the right of your typical part, and that looks like it will work.

Your thoughts often drift back to times when you got caught outside without one of your trusty baseball caps, and the wind was blowing like crazy – like the time you decided to walk across the street to lunch with friends, only to be devastated by the wind blowing your hair so much you ended up in the bathroom trying to recover your composure and hairdo. Your thoughts slowly skim over the same ground they do every morning: all the camping trips, hiking trips, swimming, and other invitations you have dodged or begged off because of your hair. You know there is no way you could join your friends on these outings and keep your hair loss a secret, plus you feel too ugly and embarrassed to be social. Your greatest fear is someone finding out about your bare spots on your scalp. So, you avoid places with mirrors and strong overhead lighting. You like softer lights that have been dimmed.

Whew! You breathe a sigh of relief, still trying to get your hair just right to cover up any gaping areas on your scalp. You absolutely don't want to be "found out" by your coworkers, friends, or worst of all, your boss. That would be far too embarrassing.

I have always had a passion and drive to help others, and that resulted in getting involved in a hair product business. Through this business, I have had the phenomenal opportunity to meet and become friends with women I likely never would have otherwise encountered.

As I shared my products, I realized I had not effectively dealt with my own hair loss. Ironically, I didn't have any idea just how bad my hair looked until I improved my hair quantity and quality and decided to look back at pictures from before I started using the products. What makes it scary is just how deep in denial I was! It wasn't until my hair started growing back in that I realized I had buried the truth deep within me. Thankfully, I began connecting to myself – and to you and your hair loss.

I know how hard it is to share with anyone that your hair is falling out. Have you even been able to convince yourself to talk to your doctor? If you have, you may have heard your concerns and struggles dismissed as "no big deal." So many of us have heard that, as well as the dismissive, "It's not life threatening."

I can't imagine hobbling into the doctor's office on crutches and wearing a full leg cast and hearing the doctor say, "Oh, it's really not a big deal. After all, it isn't life-threatening. It may or may not heal up. Be prepared to replace your leg with a transplant in a year, maybe two." I would think the doctor had lost her mind, and I would set off to find a different doctor! Yet this is what has happened to most of us who consult doctors about our hair loss.

So, I am writing this book for you. Like you, I've struggled with hair loss. And I've worked with many women who are in the same boat. Take my client Ann, for example. Little does her doctor know how depressed she is or how difficult it is for her to get up in the morning knowing she has to comb her hair, shower, and style it as best she can. Or how much hair she scoops up after her shower each day and throws in the trash. It is a part of her, and yet here she is, throwing it away by the handful. You and I know she is sobbing off and on during the process, making it take longer than ever to get ready for her day.

The few friends she has confided in have told her that they really can't tell she has lost any hair, but *she can actually see* her bare scalp in the mirror. She knows they either aren't paying any attention or are lying to her. She gets so uncomfortable when she spends any time with them.

As Ann begins pulling back from the activities she loves, others who don't know Ann, or those who haven't dealt with hair loss, may think of her as a victim, stand-offish, depressed. It may even confuse her friends who feel her pulling away and wonder if she is offended or overly sensitive. If she is outside and the wind is blowing, it will mess up her carefully styled hair, moving the strands that she spent an hour and a half painstakingly arranging this morning. You know. You have dealt with it too. None of us wants to be found out!

She wears a hat most days to protect her head from sunburn and to keep her secret. Ann shared with me her massive fear that others will find out that her hair is almost gone. Her life has become defined by her hair – well, actually, by the loss of her hair.

She knows her hair doesn't complement her appearance anymore; it has become a nuisance and a test every morning, resulting in a tremendous amount of stress for Ann as she gets ready for work. She gets up earlier and earlier as her hair keeps thinning. It is so embarrassing to her, and she just doesn't know what to do.

If your story is at all like this, you are in the right place. Keep reading. This book is for you! I mentioned earlier that, to those on the outside, my client Ann might appear to be a helpless victim. It is quite the contrary. She has used the challenge of hair loss to develop the time management skills of a ninja. She has learned to get up earlier so she can have her hair fixed before her kids and husband get up. She gets up at least two hours earlier than her family so she can shower and fix her hair. Once that is completed, she starts waking up the rest of her family and making them breakfast.

Her ninja skills include making lunches while cooking breakfast and she has learned some killer multi-tasking skills as well as shortcuts to get things prepared, served or bagged up as the case may be, and cleaned up. It is a long morning before she even gets the kids on the bus, kisses her husband goodbye and heads to work herself. She is the first to get up in the morning and the last to leave the house in the morning. Most of us would be exhausted by this time instead of just starting our work day. She has already put in two hours getting ready and a marathon 90 minutes getting her family ready to go out the door.

Imagine how much more rest Ann will get once her hair loss issues are resolved! Think about how she will feel when she learns about why she is losing hair, and how others have lost hair and gotten it back through not just temporary solutions, but one amazingly innovative solution. I can't wait for her to take the thinning hair quiz, learn her results, and get on the best path for her.

Many women think their only solutions are wearing a hat, wearing a wig, or something more invasive, like getting a hair transplant – which, by the way, is not a guaranteed method of hair regrowth. I will share with you stories of real women who have had severe hair loss and who have had amazing results, as well as those who choose to go the route of using temporary solutions. Every woman has to decide for herself which solution works best for her. No solution is for everyone, but some are more universally helpful than others. And one is more comprehensive than all the others.

Are you like Ann? She has been in some fairly stressful situations with her hair, like the time she walked across the street with her friends for lunch without remembering to check to see how much the wind might be blowing that day. After all, she lives in South Dakota, and the wind is nearly constant. Then, she went on that one retreat where the adventure day included deep-sea fishing. She could barely keep her hat on her hair, and when everyone else jumped in the water mid-afternoon to cool off, she had to pretend she wasn't feeling well and went inside to the bathroom in the cabin.

It's always tricky, and as much as she dreads these types of situations, she is very adept at reacting in a way that seems appropriate – or so she hopes. She used to really enjoy hiking, boating, camping, and swimming. She actually tries to avoid those activities now, and it has been hard coming up with reasons to give the friends that she used to accompany.

They haven't been easy to convince that she "can't" do those things anymore – she has used excuses from being allergic to the sun to heat stroke to pollen allergies to a variety of physical injuries. Her friends really aren't convinced. They just gradually stopped asking her to join them.

It has been painful for her to let those things go. She wanted to share those activities with her husband and kids. She loves nature, and it appears to be a thing of the past for her. Now she spends time indoors playing video games with her kids, knowing there is so much more they could be doing outside. She feels like she has lost a part of herself.

She has the memories of enjoying being outside and feeling free, with the wind in her hair. She can still hear some of the sounds, though the memories are fading. The smells are still there. She is afraid that she has lost that part of her forever. Oh, to have that back again. I can't wait to give Ann – and you! – The gift of a full head of hair through the resources in this book!

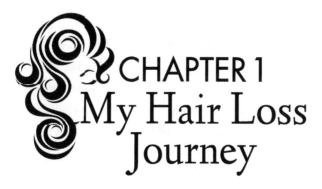

CHAPTER 1
My Hair Loss Journey

My Story

A long with the terror of being discovered by co-workers and friends and family, I also tried to keep the truth from myself at times. One of the things that is universal for women with hair loss is the denial that comes with it. I found that it was easier to put my hair loss out of my mind than it was to deal with it.

In 2014, I started losing hair. At first I thought, "Hmm, it seems like I am losing more hair in the shower, but that can't be happening so it must just seem like more than normal. This went on for a while – me not listening to myself.

At some point, I realized I was losing tons of hair. I began to dread washing it because it was coming out in ribbons. I couldn't figure out what was going on. At the same time I noticed a lot of scaly build-up on my scalp along with terrible flaking and itching. The center of my back seemed to be breaking out and itching uncontrollably. I thought I just had dry skin on my back. I like hot showers and I thought maybe I was drying out my skin. I thought somehow it was related to winter and dry air.

I had also been diagnosed with rosacea several years earlier, so I attributed most facial acne and dry skin to that. I had for a number of years been experiencing dry skin along each side of my nose and on my forehead and even into my eyebrows. Perhaps this was just some new version of rosacea, now appearing on my back?

Looking back on it now, I realize just how much denial I was in.

I went along my merry way, with flaky itching scalp, itching back, and hair coming out in ribbons, for quite some time. Eventually, I mentioned it to my medical provider, who thought it was a form of yeast infection and prescribed me some shampoo to use. I thought she really couldn't be correct. Who ever heard of a yeast infection on your head and back?!

Finally, my husband had an appointment with a dermatologist in another city since there wasn't one near our home at the time. I decided that since I was riding along for the trip (it takes us a full day to go to specialist appointments since we live in a rural state), I would make an appointment and see the dermatologist too.

When I met with the dermatologist and described my symptoms, she took a look at my skin on my face and back, as well as my scalp. She quickly diagnosed me with a severe yeast infection. I thought, *Really?! You have got to be kidding!* So, I asked her about my hair coming out. Turns out that, yes, that too is a symptom of a yeast infection on the scalp.

The worst thing she told me is that "we can manage it, but it will never completely go away." Now I knew enough about our digestive system to ask if I should change anything about my diet. I thought she would at least say to cut or limit sugar and use probiotics. Nope, she didn't say either of those things. Instead she told me that my diet was not involved and prescribed me an ointment for my skin, liquid for my scalp, a special shampoo, and oral medication, which I had to ingest one hour before I was involved in vigorous activity to the point of sweating. *Really?! I have to exercise now?*

I gave it the Girl Scout try, or so I thought, because I wanted it gone. I used the shampoo, the oral medication, and ointments. They helped, but didn't really resolve anything, and I think I just finally gave up. The easiest way for me to deal with giving up was to bury it deep within me. I just pushed all of the thoughts, feelings, and anything related to the yeast infection and hair loss deep down inside of me. Some of these feelings went so deep; I didn't even realize they were there until I started writing this book.

In reality, I just *thought* I wanted the yeast infection gone. Have you ever felt that way? It took a life coach asking me if I really wanted something to change, or if I just wanted to want something to happen for me to realize that if I had wanted it badly enough, I'd have never given up. It took slowing down a bit and listening to that a few times to really get it to sink in.

Did I want to fix my hair loss, or did I just want to want it? That is such a hard question. Ugh! It hits me deep in my being. I really thought I wanted to take care of my hair loss and yeast infection. It strikes me now just how resistant to dealing with all of that I was. I still drank soda, pop, Coke, whatever you want to call it. It really is just liquid sugar! I had known for years that

I shouldn't be drinking it. Pop wasn't the only sugar in my life, but it was my go-to sugar.

I looked at pop (in my case, Dr. Pepper) as my friend, confidante, and source of support in times of sadness, drink of celebration, pleasure giver, and the healer of all my stomach ills. As I look back and think about how educated I am and how much information is available to us in this electronic age about what we put in our bodies and the affect these things have on our systems, I am blown away by how little love and attention I gave myself. Sure, I took some steps to make sure I was doing self-care. I got a massage once a month, and I enjoyed a hobby that kept me grounded and in touch with myself. But I stopped short of truly doing what it took to heal.

Really?! Is it possible for a can of soda to be all those things? It was, because I chose to let it be all those things. You see, for me, it was safe. It can be easier to have an inanimate object as your confidante, especially if it is food of some kind, and most especially sugar. No worries about a can of soda sharing your deepest darkest secrets or your desires and aspirations. Soda definitely did not laugh at my dreams and tell me I could never accomplish them. Soda did not say to me, "I knew you wouldn't finish that project," or, "What made you think you could make money serving others? It's wrong to make money serving others."

I also know that soda was no friend of mine and absolutely not a healer. Those are stories I told myself for over 40 years. How could a friend or healer damage my body the way a can of soda can? The acid ate away at my teeth, and damaged my digestive system. The sugar caused inflammation in every organ and system in my body AND exacerbated my hair loss! It was time to get real, truly real, and deal with the root causes of my pop addiction and dependence. Ugh! I had no choice if I was going to serve others.

What about you? What is the root cause of your hair loss? Have you dealt with it, or do you simply *want to want* to deal with it? I am not saying Dr. Pepper was the sole cause of my hair loss. The root cause was much deeper within me, and I chose to deal with it by drinking Dr. Pepper, adding significantly to my sugar intake, which then helped feed the yeast infection. Had I dealt with my emotional needs to begin with instead of burying them, I may never have experienced hair loss.

Where Do I Begin?

I knew exactly what I needed to do to deal with my pop issue. I journaled my thoughts and feelings and began sharing my experience with others like you. That allowed me to process it mentally and emotionally.

I also have learned so much about myself through journaling. It is ironic to me that I still sometimes resist journaling, but as soon as I sit down with a pretty notebook and my pen, the words just spill out. Journaling is a way for us women to process things. We tend to hang on to things because we don't know how to process them.

For women, speaking our thoughts and feelings in a safe environment and journaling them are effective methods to process what we bury on the inside. I know that, without these tools, I would not have been able to walk my way through my reasons for drinking Dr. Pepper. I know it isn't a big deal to be addicted to pop in most people's eyes. But I realize I was using it as a means of burying my thoughts and feelings.

Knowing how to deal with my issues is the craziest, most awesome feeling in the world. I know God is on this journey with me, and He alone put me on this path to freedom and solving my hair loss issue and yours too! Learn how to deal with issues instead of burying them under a pile of pop cans, and your self-assurance will soar!

The Rest of the Story

Are you ready to get that spring back in your step? We're coming to that part. Let's get back to my story and finish it before we move on. I don't know about you, but I used to love listening to Paul Harvey's stories and, in particular, his "Rest of the Story" segments. Here is my "Rest of the Story" segment: I would have continued on with terrible hair (I had no true idea of how bad it had actually gotten) had God not divinely connected me, through a series of circumstances, to my ultimate hair solution. In September of 2016, I traveled to southeastern Oklahoma to visit my dad and other family. It's a 1000-mile trip one-way, and not practical to fly because each of us is located hours from major airports. I have gotten to where I spend a substantial amount of time at my destination after driving that far. So I was at my dad's house for a couple of weeks.

While I was at my dad's house, my cousin's daughter, Rebecca, invited me to an event she was hosting at her salon in town. I had been seeing some social media posts about some new company she was in and a product she was selling. To be honest, I really hadn't paid attention because it seemed my Facebook newsfeed had been inundated from similar posts from lots of my friends.

I decided I would go support her since I had been in similar companies, and knew it sometimes is a challenge to get guests to come to events like the one she was hosting. When I arrived, no one else was there yet, and it gave me a chance to ask her specific questions. I really pressed her about why she had joined this company and about the products. She answered all my questions and then started sharing her results and the results of others using the products.

When I saw her before and after picture and learned about the company culture and how well the company and its products had already been received, I was encouraged. She sent me back to my dad's with samples in hand, which I tried that night. I truly liked how my hair felt after using the products. The most ironic thing was that when she told me about the hair regrowth ingredient in the products, I immediately thought "my husband could really use this." I was still in so much denial I never really thought about my own hair loss or other women who may be experiencing hair loss.

After trying the samples and reading as much material as I could on the website, I too joined the company. My thoughts were, *if these products can help Rebecca's hair in such a profound way and are so well-received by customers, then I want to be a part of it. And, my husband may be able to grow his hair back!* I will share more in a later chapter about the actual product and its active ingredients.

I began using the products right away and sharing them with my friends. I wanted to share them with everyone because they had so much potential. As time went on, I helped one of my new business partners with her business launch. I remember it well. It was the Sunday after Thanksgiving, and we had driven all the way home from a family celebration in Wisconsin. My husband and daughter weren't too happy that I needed to be home by a specific time, but they supported me anyway.

I had invited a couple of my friends who I had known for 12 years, but hadn't seen in the three months prior. My friends came to the launch, and some of the business partner's guests were there too. The creepy thing was that my friends stared at me the entire time I was sharing information during the presentation. I was uncomfortable.

Finally, one of my friends blurted out, "I can't quit staring at your hair, Myrna." She proceeded to tell me that my hair was so much better than the last time she had seen me, she couldn't believe it. My hair was filling in, and I had barely realized it. Then again, I was the person who was unaware of how bad my hair had looked before using these products.

My two friends joined me in the business a week later, and as soon as one of their aunts saw my hair at their launch, she signed up as a preferred customer. Their family deals with hair loss and has two members dealing with cancer and the results of chemotherapy on their hair. Another friend has lupus and takes medication that causes her hair to break off and fall out. She had lost a lot of hair, and had been trying other products with no results. We were all excited at the prospect of the results we could experience.

Then, near the end of December, I posted a live video on my Facebook page about my hair having more volume. One of the ladies who responded and requested more information lived in the northeastern part of South Dakota. When I talked with her over the phone she sounded so skeptical and even angry that I wasn't sure what to expect. She told me she had tried every product she could find, and that this product was her last option before having hair sewn into her scalp.

She reluctantly placed an order with me, and then I didn't hear a peep out of her for a month. Exactly one month from the day she started using these products, she posted before and after pictures that were remarkable! I believed in the products and knew they could help, but I had no idea what they could truly do until then. I had the pleasure of meeting this lady a few months later and was blown away by her gratitude. That was the best day ever!

That was the day and the reason I became so passionate about helping women with hair loss. Are you ready for this ride? Are you ready to do something for yourself? Let's go!

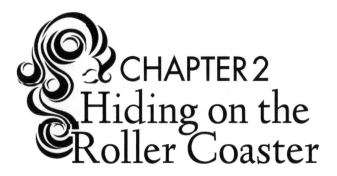

CHAPTER 2
Hiding on the
Roller Coaster

Planning and Preparing

You absolutely don't want to be "found out" by your coworkers, friends, or of all people, your boss. Just thinking about your boss and coworkers finding out about your balding head rattles you to the core. You start trembling, then something clicks and you realize this is not what you want to be thinking about or dwelling on any more. In fact, you want to find positive things to think about and listen to, since it really sets you up for a much better day. It is a daily challenge to keep your thoughts off your hair – or the lack of it.

You remember clearly the first day in the shower when you experienced what felt and looked like handfuls of hair falling out. You could not believe you were holding your hair in your hands and that it was actually no longer attached to your head. You were so confused, and the words in your mind kept going in circles: "Am I losing my hair? Why is my hair coming out in big blobs in my hand? Is that really my hair in my hands? I'm not losing my hair. Women don't lose their hair. This is a bad dream and I will wake up soon. Am I losing my hair?" Round and round your brain went, even as you were drying off. You knew you had to look in the mirror, but you were afraid of what you were going to see and how you were going to respond if this wasn't a bad dream.

It took you a few days to get over the initial shock of that image in the mirror that first day. After taking a few days off work to get an ounce of control over your emotions and to figure out your best options for disguising your hair loss, you fell into a routine. It wasn't a routine that you wanted, that's for sure. It includes you getting up two hours earlier just to make yourself what you feel is presentable.

You bought a wardrobe of caps and hats to match the outfits you already owned, and you spent time trying different hair styles and researching hair loss in women. The information you found was confusing and overwhelming since there are so many different causes of hair loss. You had no idea that 40% of those suffering from hair loss were women! That is over 21 million (21,000,000) women just like you. You wondered where these women were hiding.

Then, you began the steep climb up the roller coaster track when you encountered your first challenging circumstance: you walked across the street with your friends for lunch, never even thinking of the wind that was blowing that day. You ended up in the bathroom instead of eating lunch because your hair had been whipped all over the place and you were just sure your friends had seen, it, you know, your bald spot. It felt just like being on that rollercoaster hanging almost upside down going up that first steep incline. You felt like you had no control over the situation and helpless. That was really a rough day. You were so embarrassed and emotional.

Then, another time you and your family were visiting relatives and the group decided to grill at the park. The day was beautiful, the park was green and next to the river, and you had your husband and kids with you. Everything was perfect – well almost. You were so preoccupied by thoughts of your hair and wondering if the wind was going to start blowing and reveal your bare scalp that you really didn't enjoy the day. You never thought to throw in some of your ball caps because you weren't quite in the habit of thinking through every little detail just yet. By the end of the day, you were angry at your family for wanting to go to the park; wait, no, you were really angry at yourself for forgetting to bring a hat, and you were also angry at the situation. Ugh! Why was this hair loss thing plaguing you?

Learning to Adapt

After the park incident, you quickly learned to adapt to unexpected and challenging circumstances. Talk about developing skills – after learning to adapt, you could be a trainer for your company on being flexible and making the most of your circumstances! Once you began adapting to challenging circumstances by planning ahead and learning to make quick decisions, you felt the roller coaster pause at the top of the track. You recognized the feeling from times you had ridden the roller coaster at the state fair long before you started losing your hair. It was a feeling of anxiety, nervous anticipation that comes just before the roller coaster plunges down the other side. You began feeling more and more alone and less like a woman. It caused that same sick feeling in your stomach just like being at the top of the roller coaster. As you plunged down the other side, you felt depression creeping in and trying to take up residence. Fortunately you realized what was happening and decided you would not, could not, let that happen.

Choosing Your Emotional Path

You had seen depression take over others' lives and you did not want to go down that path, so you started looking for a solution – really an alternative. You wanted something, someplace where you could learn options, a place to seek guidance from those who already dealt with hair loss; a place where you felt safe to learn to be you again. You no longer wanted to be "that woman with the balding head." You wanted to solve your hair loss problem so you could be spontaneous again – at least if that was possible. You really didn't know if it was possible, but you wanted to find out. You had never been a victim and you decided you didn't want to start now.

Learning from Others

You did some internet searches and found a couple of great groups that support women just like you. You started following the posts and asking questions. You found stories from women like Ruth; Ruth noticed thinning for a bit. In March she found the bald spots on one side of her head. Her general practitioner was insensitive and pretty much worthless. So, she referred herself to a dermatologist but they had no appointments for over a month. The results from the blood tests she strongly requested the general practitioner do after she did some research about them were all normal. Now it is April, two weeks out from her appointment still, and the bald patches and thinning are spreading across her head. She is losing her pretty long curls... she wants to hide. She's so depressed! She can barely wait another two weeks! And that's just to see them for the first time. It all feels so hopeless for Ruth.

You read about Sherry, whose hair fell out after illness about a year ago. She wrote that she no longer looks like a scalped scarecrow, but her hair is still hideously short and she realizes she has been depressed about her hair for an entire year. She hates herself so much she says she can't even cry about it anymore. She is unemployed and relies on her family for money. She is too tired to live and too tired to die. While she is glad some of her hair grew back, she is disappointed because what little came back is 95 percent grey and extremely coarse. She can't even bring herself to leave her home. It was heart-wrenching to read this post; because you understand and at the same time, fear this may be you down the road.

Then you read Anita's post, which you really identified with, despite the fact that she is a blonde and you have long, flowing black hair – or used to. Anita had been suffering from unexplained hair loss for the past year. It had started unexpectedly last November. She is a natural blonde, so she already had thin hair. She noticed that she lost the most hair when it was wet, so she told herself she would only wash it every other day to avoid the trauma of seeing all the hair loss. That was a sacrifice for her, since she has oily hair. She started embracing her natural wave and tried to keep it as natural as possible. The loss continued, which resulted in a doctor's appointment. Everything came back normal, so she did some research and asked to have her ferritin level tested. Her doctor refused, so she did it on her own. It came back low, but not low enough to be recognized as an issue, so she gave up. She truly believes there is something wrong medically, but no one wants to help.

You become engrossed in the stories and read a few each night after work, trying not to be pulled in emotionally and yet

... you want to know more – you want to know if these women have their hair back yet.

How Many Women Share Your Hair Loss Nightmare?

More than you might think. According to the American Academy of Dermatology, "Forty percent of *women have* visible *hair loss* by the time they are age 40." (Emphasis mine.) That is almost half of all women! If you're like me, you're thinking there has got to be a better way to deal with hair loss. You have seen other women just like you who are suffering emotionally, physically, relationally, and financially all because of hair loss. It really is a nightmare for the women you have read about, and you're probably starting to feel that it is for you, too. You feel indignant and just plain mad that more hasn't been done to help women with hair loss, much less prepare women for this huge change in their lives.

Why is it that it seems so much more acceptable for men to have thinning hair and be bald than it is for women? And why, oh why hasn't someone come up with something that works?! You also wonder why some in the medical community don't seem to understand hair loss in women and many don't seem to care. Wow! Changes need to be made! You decide you want to learn more about the causes of hair loss in women and find a better way to deal with it.

CHAPTER 3
What Is Causing Your Hair Loss?

Three Key Concepts

There are three key concepts I have learned along the way. One of the most important is that hair loss in women is a complex issue often caused by underlying medical conditions. The second key concept is that one type of treatment may work for one person and not the next. And the third key concept is that every woman deals with hair loss differently. Let's look at each of those.

Key Concept 1

Hair loss in women is a complex issue often caused by underlying medical conditions. What are some of the underlying medical issues than can result in hair loss? It seems that by and large they are related to changes in hormones ... are you surprised? Some of the underlying conditions include ovarian cysts, high-androgen index birth control pills, pregnancy, menopause, thyroid issues, and poly-cystic ovarian syndrome (PCOS).

Hormone balance in women is a thing and should be addressed jointly with your medical practitioner. Once you are managing the underlying cause, you give yourself a much better chance of re-growing your hair. You can get started on a path to re-growing your hair, but without a diagnosis and treatment plan of the internal body, you will most likely be fighting a losing battle.

Dihydrotestosterone (DHT) is a derivative of the male hormone testosterone. DHT is at the root of multiple types of hair loss including androgenetic alopecia. DHT is attracted to an enzyme that is held in a hair follicle's oil glands. In essence, it shrinks the hair follicles, making it impossible for them to survive. If we can block DHT, we can prevent hair loss and minimize damage done to the hair follicles.

Interestingly, DHT occurs in both men and women. For women, when female hormones are lowered, it tips the balance in favor of the male hormones (androgens) like DHT. That, as well as in a host of other medical issues, is when hair loss occurs.

The American Hair Loss Association has this to say: "Hormones are cyclical. Testosterone levels in some men drop by 10 percent each decade after thirty. Women's hormone levels decline as menopause approaches and drop sharply during menopause and beyond. The cyclic nature of both our hair and hormones is one reason hair loss can increase in the short term even when you are experiencing a long-term slowdown of hair loss (and a long-term increase in hair growth) while on a treatment that controls hair loss."

Key Concept 2

One type of treatment may work for one person and not the next. In addition to working with my clients, I have been interviewing women with hair loss and observing women's hair loss forums, and one of the most prevalent comments I have heard and seen is that hair loss treatment is not a one-size-fits-all proposition. I also found that women feel unheard and disrespected in this area by the medical profession and sales representatives.

It is important to keep this in mind when trying hair loss treatments. If you have followed the instructions and used it the suggested length of time and it doesn't work for you, try something else. Exhaust your options. I have some suggested treatment options in this book in Chapter Four. Also, check out Chapter Five where I share stories of women with hair loss, causes and what worked for them. The biggest issues I have seen are not following the usage instructions correctly and not getting to the root of the problem (the underlying issues).

Key Concept 3

Every woman deals with hair loss differently. One woman may try every possible treatment before resorting to a wig, while another may try one option or none and then move toward a wig. There are some high-quality wigs out there that really help women like you feel like yourself again as much as you can short of having your own hair. I realize having your own hair grow back is the ultimate goal, and my wish is for you to have that if at all possible.

One thing that is universal is the emotional toll hair loss takes on women. Most women like you describe serious depression and difficulty getting out of bed in the morning.

They can't bear to comb their hair or wash it because they know they will have handfuls of hair come out. It is devastating to you, making it difficult to not only enjoy but participate in everyday life.

In what seems like an evil twist, you learn that the antidepressants prescribed by your doctor cause ... you guessed it: hair loss! It seems hair loss is lurking around every corner, and the medical community is more often than not dismissive. I am not surprised you are depressed and don't want to tell anyone. My purpose in this book is to empower you and to let you know, you are not alone. There are more than 21 million of us here with you. I also want to share a comprehensive solution with you that is different than the other options you have been given up to now. Let's talk about causes of hair loss now and start finding answers for you.

Causes of Hair Loss

I find if I have an issue or challenge, the more I know about it, the more prepared I am to face it head on. That is why I am including descriptions of the different causes of hair loss and writing them in terms everyone can understand. I don't know about you, but I get turned off by overly technical or scientific terms. When I was doing my own research, every description I read was highly technical and difficult to understand. I learned when I was in school that if I could break down the technical/ scientific type mumbo jumbo, I could understand it better, and so that is what I have done for you here. I hope you find it helpful and that the descriptions help you meet your hair loss head on (no pun intended).

Alopecia

Alopecia is the general term for hair loss. It sounds like this big, scary word and that is how we use it, but it really means HAIR LOSS on any part of the body, nothing more. Let's take away the power we have given this word and start thinking "hair loss" when we hear it so that we can begin to empower ourselves to take control of our situations.

Androgenic/Androgenetic Alopecia

Androgenic Alopecia is also known as Male/Female Pattern Baldness. This refers to a male hormone, androgen, that is present in small amounts in women. Most women with this type of hair loss also have an underlying condition related to hormones. Remember what I said about DHT earlier? It is thought to be the main culprit in this type of hair loss. The delicate hormonal balance gets out of whack so that you end up with a higher amount of the male hormone than female hormone. That's when DHT affects your hair follicles. You may have Poly-cystic Ovarian Syndrome (PCOS), or ovarian cysts, or you may take birth control pills that are high on the androgen index. You may be or have been pregnant, in menopause, or dealing with thyroid issues. Each of these can play a role in female pattern baldness.

Telogen Effluvium

Telogen Effluvium relates to a specific phase that hair is in when it sheds or falls out in high numbers. Telogen is the resting phase of your hair – it is the third and final phase of the hair cycle. Effluvium means an unpleasant discharge. This type of hair loss is typically the result of your body going through a traumatic event like childbirth, malnutrition, a severe infection, major surgery, or extreme stress. And it affects 6 to 8 percent of your hair. One woman reported that her hair loss occurred after she quit smoking. It generally occurs six weeks to three months after the traumatic event – just when you think things are back to normal and you have no worries.

Anagen Effluvium

Anagen Effluvium also relates to a specific phase the hair is in when it is affected and sheds. Anagen is the active phase of the hair, when hair follicle cells are rapidly dividing and growing. This type of hair loss occurs when there has been an impact to the hair follicle that affects the division of the nucleus or the metabolism of the cells. This is typically caused by chemotherapy, which is designed to strategically target rapidly dividing cancer cells in the body. Since hair follicle cells are also rapidly dividing, they are often greatly affected by chemotherapy. Thankfully, this type of hair loss is not typically permanent and your hair will regrow after chemotherapy is completed. Use quality hair products the entire time you are on chemo and set yourself up for the best possible hair regrowth when chemo is finished. There are some great options for you in a later chapter.

Traction Alopecia

Traction Alopecia is hair loss caused by localized trauma or stress to the hair follicles, often from tight hairstyles like tight ponytails, cornrows, braids, and extensions. Traction means the action of drawing or pulling a thing over a surface. The hair is pulled taut in these hair styles, stressing the follicle over time.

Basically, if you are always putting your hair in a tight ponytail, bun or braid, it will likely break off eventually. The best way to prevent this is to alternate how you wear your hair so that it isn't always tightly pulled back. If you are in a job where you need to wear your hair pulled back, let your hair down as soon as you get home to give it a rest and use products that will strengthen the hair follicle and shaft.

Medications

Many of the medications we take to treat illnesses and chronic conditions like lupus and seizure disorders actually MAKE OUR HAIR FALL OUT as a side effect. It seems so unfair and like an endless cycle. You have an illness or chronic condition like lupus, like my friend Geli; you are prescribed chemotherapy drugs to manage your lupus; and your hair starts breaking and falling out, leaving big wads of hair in the shower and broken pieces of hair in the sink after you get ready for work in the morning. Then, you become depressed, are prescribed an antidepressant, and your hair falls out even more! You've seen the doctor multiple times in the cycle only for him/her to say, "At least you still have some hair. It's not life-threatening." I understand why it seems so hopeless and why you just want to lock yourself away.

Your doctor may not mention hair loss as a side effect of some drugs, so don't forget to do your own research and read the drug manufacturers' complete warnings. Your pharmacist can provide you with this information even before you fill a prescription. Many pill and medication guidebooks (sold in bookstores and pharmacies) are also excellent sources of complete information about prescription drugs. If your doctor prescribes medications to treat depression, epilepsy, lupus, or heart disease, ask if one that does not have hair loss as a possible side effect can be substituted. Examples of medications that can cause hair loss include trimethadione used to treat epilepsy; Prozac (fluoxetine hydrochloride) used to treat depression; and beta blockers used to treat glaucoma and high blood pressure. A chart of medications that may also cause hair loss is included in the appendix.

Some of my clients have gone to great lengths to find out what is causing their hair loss only to be told by their medical practitioner that they don't know why it is falling out. I am sure you can quickly identify with the devastation that kind of a non-diagnosis presents. Take Elaine, as she has gotten older, her hair has gotten thinner. She has always had downy soft, baby fine hair, so, when it thins, it is devastating. She doesn't know what to do and in her way thinks it is just part of the aging process.

And that could be the case. But when you take a look at the causes of hair loss, age doesn't even make an appearance. Elaine is on medications for everything under the sun, but when she asks her doctor about it, her doctor quickly dismisses her hair loss as no big deal, telling her not to worry about it since she still has hair. She is left with no answers, and no idea that it could be menopause, medications, stress, or other issues that are causing her to lose her hair.

No diagnosis is the most challenging "diagnosis" of all. And then add to that being dismissed by the doctor as over-reacting. For women, losing their hair can be particularly devastating. Of course what the medical community doesn't seem to realize is that the psychological damage caused by hair loss and feeling unattractive can be just as devastating as any serious disease, and, in fact, can take an emotional toll that directly affects physical health. Hair loss is a serious life altering issue.

As you are navigating the waters of your hair loss journey, remember the three key concepts I mentioned at the beginning of this chapter: hair loss in women is a complex issue often caused by underlying medical conditions; one type of treatment may work for one person and not the next; and every woman deals with hair loss differently. Chapter Four and will give you the information you need to help you move toward dealing with your hair loss and re-growing as much as you can. Chapter Six describes a comprehensive approach to help you find the underlying cause(s) and resolve your hair loss.

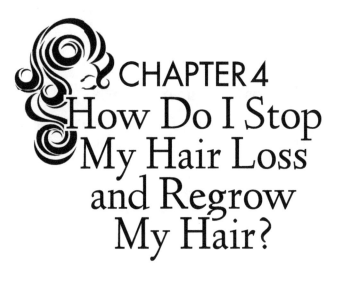

CHAPTER 4
How Do I Stop My Hair Loss and Regrow My Hair?

Background

I have shared with you the numerous potential causes for your hair loss and now I want to give you practical solutions to resolve your hair loss as quickly as possible. As mentioned earlier, this is not a one-size-fits-all solution. You most likely will need a combination of these solutions as you travel on your journey. From my experience personally and with my clients, the comprehensive approach in Chapter Six is what will give you the best possible outcome.

Hair Loss Dollars and Sense

According to Niche Hacks (http://nichehacks.com/hair-loss-niche-report/), 56 million people, including 21 million women in the US alone, are losing their hair and spending $4 billion trying to get it back. Hair loss is emotionally distressing, which makes those afflicted particularly vulnerable to an industry that includes charlatans ready to take advantage of those dealing with hair loss. I have seen the distrust and skepticism of hair regrowth products in my clients, and it is understandable. Unfortunately, those who have been taken advantage of may not be willing to try innovative products that appear on the market, therefore, short-changing themselves on potential hair regrowth. My hope is that this book helps you sort through the information so that you can make the best decision for yourself.

Consider the Side Effects

There have been a number of treatments on the market for some time including medications, hair and scalp treatments, and supplements. The medications often come with side effects and do not always work, plus you are adding additional chemicals to your body. For instance, this is what one site said about one medication specifically used for hair regrowth: "When applied to the scalp, it often stimulates hair growth. The *exact way it works is not known* [emphasis mine], but it is thought to improve the blood flow around the hair follicle and stimulate the hair follicle to grow hair."

I don't know about you, but I want to know how and why certain products work, especially if they are harsh chemicals that can do things like age my skin and affect my blood pressure. And this product is actually approved by the Food and Drug Administration (FDA). Really?! I can't imagine why they would approve something like that – they are supposed to be protecting the US public! And it is the only one endorsed by the American Hair Loss Association because it is approved by the FDA.

I am absolutely shocked that these organizations, who are supposed to be protecting and guiding us, are approving and endorsing something like this. It originally was developed as a blood pressure medication and now it is for hair regrowth?! Women and men with hair loss should not accept that sort of help.

In addition, of the women I know who have tried this particular medication, almost all said it did not work or that they didn't use it long enough because of the effect it had on the hair they had left. I have included the potential side effects of this product below. Look it over and decide for yourself if this is what you want to be exposed to daily.

Potential Side Effects:

- Burning of the scalp
- Changes in blood pressure
- Dizziness
- Feeling faint
- Headache
- Inflammation or soreness at the hair root
- Persistent local rash

(Med Broadcast Website)

Many of those using topical treatments report experiencing side effects. One woman reported that it noticeably aged the skin on her face. It usually takes six or more months of use for the medication to work. Hair may fall out when *it* is first used. This is a temporary effect of the medication. *Important: once hair starts to grow, it will stay for as long as the medication is used. The hair will begin to fall out again a few months after the applications are stopped.* I added the italics for emphasis because I want you to let this sink in. You have to keep using the product once you start or your hair will fall out again!

I recommend and urge that you carefully read the labels and research the side effects of the included ingredients of any product you put in or on your scalp.

Ways to Temporarily Disguise Your Hair Loss

While you are waiting for your hair to grow back in, there are some things you can do to disguise your hair loss. Some of them are: products that add volume to your hair, colored fibers that mimic the look of hair, scalp tinting/coloring products like scalp powder, wigs, hair pieces, extensions, and the style of your cut.

Volumizing Products

Volumizing products are great! The volumizing products I use actually enlarge the hair follicle, making it look and feel like you have more hair. Not only that, they *are naturally based with no harsh chemicals*! That is important to me, and I bet it is to you, too.

I strictly used volumizing products for the first 11 months. I loved how they made my hair feel and look. It was like I had more hair right away because of their properties. My hair needed the volume! Now I use a hydrating shampoo and volumizing conditioner for the best possible combination. The hydration shampoo enhances my curls while the conditioner gives me volume. Choosing the right products for you is important when you have hair loss. Typically, a company consultant can help you decide the best products for your current hair condition. Keep in mind that you may need to change products down the road as your hair condition improves.

Colored Fibers and Tints to Mimic Your Hair Color

These may be actual hair or other fibers that are colored similar to your hair color. The ladies I know who have used the fibers didn't care for them because of the mess they made when applied and then also on their pillow at night. The fibers are effective, they are just a mess to apply and manage.

There are also products that can be used to tint your actual scalp so it appears that you have more hair than you actually do. They come in powder form, spray and lotions. Those using these products were quite satisfied with them and found them less messy than the fibers. I heard positive feedback from the ladies using these products.

Wigs, Hair Pieces, and Extensions

Wigs come in every shape, size, and color imaginable. They are made of human hair or synthetic fibers, and can be hot to wear. They can be custom-fitted for your head, and they are a great back-up plan or alternative if your hair absolutely will not grow back. You can spend as little or as much as you want on wigs. The sky is the limit.

Hair pieces and toppers can be quite useful for those with hair loss on the top. Extensions may prove useful if your hair loss is on the sides or back, but aren't viable options for hair loss on the top. Do your research to find an experienced cosmetologist to apply your extensions. Micro-bead extensions are the best option if your hair is fine and breaking. Be careful: clip-in and other types of extensions can damage what little hair you have left.

One woman I know uses micro-bead extensions to disguise her hair loss, and says she gets adjustments about every six weeks. She says the initial cost and maintenance is expensive and completely worth the investment. She spent quite a bit of time researching salons and stylists in her area before taking the leap.

Head Coverings

Hats, caps, and scarves are also useful to disguise hair loss. Get creative with them, coordinating them with your clothes, shoes, and purse. Embrace this option when you use it – choose to make it fun and enjoyable.

Creative Hairstyles

Hairstyles can also disguise thinning hair. Work with your hair stylist/cosmetologist to find a hairstyle that works best for you. And have a little fun with it! The more ways we can embrace challenges and make them fun, the less overwhelming they are. Some specific ideas, with photos, are at the end of this chapter.

A New Innovative Option

Remember the story I told you about my hair loss and regrowth back in Chapter One? Now I will share the active ingredients and the product my clients and I have been using with great results. When I was first introduced to these revolutionary products in September, 2016, I loved how they made my hair feel and look. I never even considered that the hair I had lost two years prior from the yeast infection could regrow. Amazingly, 11 months later, my hair has completely regrown and I have more hair than I ever remember having in my life. Until now, I have always had fine, thin hair. Now, I have a headful of fine hair. I have naturally curly hair, and the curls are softer and more manageable than ever.

The products I am referring to are naturally based and produced by a company named Monat Global. Monat stands for Modern Nature, and is an anti-aging hair care company offering naturally-based products. Just thinking about the difference between a product that is naturally based vs. one that was actually developed as a medication for blood pressure gives me a huge amount of peace of mind. I don't worry about putting Monat on my scalp.

Monat has created a new market segment thanks to the anti-aging component of the products. Monat doesn't try to change buying habits because we are all using hair products already. Instead they added products to meet our needs, like for hair loss and regrowth and chemically damaged hair; and then they developed products for every hair type.

The founders of Monat recognized the importance of providing products that have the science and technology behind them to meet the needs of their customers. Monat owns its own research and development lab and manufacturing facility in Miami, Florida, giving the company complete control of the products from beginning to end. All of Monat's products are produced in the US.

What Makes Monat Products *Unique?*

The simplest answer is *Rejuveniqe Oil Intensive* (fondly referred to as liquid gold by my team and me). It is an amazing product that we each love and use daily. Most women rely on an arsenal of high-end shampoos, conditioners, treatments, and creams to replace the natural oils in our scalp that get essentially stripped away every time we wash. The problem is, many of the products available lie on top of the hair and only temporarily help, assuming they help at all. Oil is vital for healthy hair and skin. Natural oil also contains antioxidants for healthy hair.

And here is what makes Monat different: Rejuveniqe Oil Intensive is infused into all but two of the products, which just happen to be water-based. When you combine this powerful oil infusion with a complete haircare line for cleansing, conditioning, hydrating, styling, and promoting healthy hair, that is uber-conscientious to avoid harmful chemicals, you've got yourself a healthier alternative *that benefits your body as well as the appearance of your hair*.

The Rejuveniqe Oil has at least 100 uses that include your skin, nails, and hair. Some favorite uses for me include adding a drop or two to my mascara to keep it from getting dry and cakey; applying it to my dry, calloused elbows – it is the only thing that will soften them up; adding a drop or two to my hair products to enhance their properties and encourage hair growth as much as possible; and putting it on my lips when I go to bed to keep them from drying out and getting chapped. Those are a few of my favorites. Here are more for you to try:

- **Pre-Shampoo Treatment** – apply a generous amount to dry or damp hair and scalp. Leave it on for 15 minutes; rinse thoroughly. Shampoo and condition as usual.

- **Intensive Hydrating Treatment** – Apply a generous amount to damp hair and scalp. Place a warm moist towel around the head and leave in for 30 minutes. Rinse thoroughly; shampoo and condition.

- **Leave-In Finishing Treatment** – Apply a small amount to hair, concentrating on the ends. Style as usual.

- **Anti-Frizz Treatment** – Rub a small amount between hands and apply to hair, concentrating on the ends. Style as usual.

- **Added Nutrition, Protection, & Shine** – Mix a pea size amount with conditioner or masque before applying.

- **Facial Moisturizer** – Apply morning and evening to face, neck and décolletage prior to moisturizer, concentrating on problem areas such as fine lines and wrinkles for instant hydration, protection, improved texture, and tone.

- Great for all areas of the body that are prone to dryness such as cuticles, nails, elbows, knees, and heels.

Don't you wonder what makes Rejuveniqe so special? I did, and I was thrilled by what I learned. It's a combination of 11 different essential oils that offer vitamins, minerals, antioxidants, beta-carotene, omega-3, fatty acids, nutrients, and amino acids. The base is Abyssinian oil. Monat chose Abyssinian oil not only for its remarkable rejuvenating properties, but also because of the way it is grown and processed. It is a rare and unique combination of fatty acids prized for their ability to do everything from mimicking the effects of silicon for unbeatable shine to lubricating the hair deep into the follicle and protecting and coating each strand.

It has a unique molecular structure not found in any other naturally occurring oil, and is enhanced with 10 other botanical oils from all over the world. Abyssinian oil increases the manageability, shine, and strength of the hair. Its molecular structure makes it biologically preferred and highly conditioning for skin and hair.

Abyssinian Oil is 100% pure vegetable oil, light, non-greasy, and easily absorbed. (It goes to work right away and doesn't sit on top of our skin like some ingredients.) It is safe and environmentally friendly since it is non-GMO, biodegradable, never tested on animals, and pure unadulterated vegetable oil. It is highly stable and resistant to oxidation and degradation with a high benefit/cost ratio.

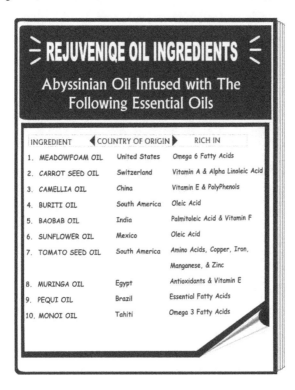

REJUVENIQE OIL INGREDIENTS

Abyssinian Oil Infused with The Following Essential Oils

INGREDIENT	COUNTRY OF ORIGIN	RICH IN
1. MEADOWFOAM OIL	United States	Omega 6 Fatty Acids
2. CARROT SEED OIL	Switzerland	Vitamin A & Alpha Linoleic Acid
3. CAMELLIA OIL	China	Vitamin E & PolyPhenols
4. BURITI OIL	South America	Oleic Acid
5. BAOBAB OIL	India	Palmitoleic Acid & Vitamin F
6. SUNFLOWER OIL	Mexico	Oleic Acid
7. TOMATO SEED OIL	South America	Amino Acids, Copper, Iron, Manganese, & Zinc
8. MURINGA OIL	Egypt	Antioxidants & Vitamin E
9. PEQUI OIL	Brazil	Essential Fatty Acids
10. MONOI OIL	Tahiti	Omega 3 Fatty Acids

The Key Ingredients in Monat's Products

The key ingredients in Monat's products are scientific terms that are not easy to say or understand. So I will share with you what they do for you and your hair:

1. Procataline helps maintain healthy levels of antioxidants in follicles to combat premature thinning while protecting color and shine. It adds nutrients to keep your hair healthy and prevent thinning.

2. Capixyl helps reduce scalp inflammation and strengthens and thickens hair while stimulating natural growth. This is the ingredient you want to be certain is in your products when you have thinning hair.

3. Rejuveniqe Oil Intensive is Monat's own proprietary blend of unique oils that contain essential and powerfully active botanical ingredients. This is the oil I described above. It contributes nutrients to develop and maintain healthy hair.

4. Crodasorb is a UV absorber that helps protect the hair from sun damage. This is the ingredient that makes Monat's products anti-aging.

Clinical Results

One of the best things about Monat is that it has clinically proven ingredients. In other words, there is no guessing what the products are capable of because they have been tested in a controlled setting by an independent lab. Remember that product I mentioned earlier where they weren't quite sure why it might work? Monat is different. Below are the things you can count on with Monat. People were in the clinical tests and this is what they reported:

- 88 out of 100 people said their hair had increased manageability and shine

- 76 out of 100 people had an increase in collagen, directly increasing follicle size

- 70 out of 100 people had an increase in repair effect, improving hair anchoring (that means the roots are stronger, which is what we want for thinning hair)

- 58 out of 100 people saw a decrease in fiber breakage (less hair in the sink)

- 48 out of 100 people saw a decrease in the DHT hormone that contributes to hair loss – this is what makes me happy! Almost half of the people had a decrease in the hormone that likes to kill our hair follicles.

- 46 out of 100 people had an increase in hair growth

- 5 out of 100 people had an increase in hair follicle strength

On top of that, Monat's products *do not contain:*

- **Phthalates** – are mainly used in plasticizers (substances added to plastics to increase their flexibility, transparency, durability, and longevity.)

- **PEG** – or poly-ethylene glycol, a thick, sticky liquid used to deliver ingredients to the skin or hair.

- **DEA/MEA** – ethanolamine compounds are found in many consumer products ranging from cosmetics, personal care products, and household cleaning products—concerns are cancer, environmental concerns.

- **Sulfates** – used as a surfactant, a mixture of molecules that can attract both water and oil. It allows soaps and shampoos to separate dirt and oil from your skin or hair and then allows the water you rinse it with to carry it off your body and down the drain. Sulfates can be irritating. The properties that allow them to carry away dirt can also strip away our natural oils.

- **Parabens** – are preservatives and found in a wide variety of personal care products. They contain estrogen-mimicking properties that are associated with increased risk of breast cancer. They are absorbed through the skin.

- **Harsh salt systems** – often used as a preservative and surfactant. These products are skin and eye irritants.

- **Harmful colors** – colors and dyes are often made with synthetic materials. Synthetic materials are manufactured, not natural, and many have been reported to be toxic.

- **Harmful fragrances** – According to the Environmental Working Group, fragrance mixes have been associated with allergies, dermatitis, respiratory distress and potential effects on the reproductive system.

Okay, I know that was a lot of mumbo jumbo. Let me break it down for you. When examining the Monat products, you'll see that they include Capixyl – except the two men's shave products – the cream shave and the aftershave + moisturizer – as well as the dry shampoo, the nutritional supplement, and the children's product line. I was really excited to learn that every product I use, except the dry shampoo, encourages hair regrowth, including the hair spray! I use the root lifter, mousse, hair spray, styling taffy and a recent addition, the curl cream, regularly. How cool is that?!

For me, that is the best possible option.

I have had personal results and seen the results of others after using these products. My client, Frances, was diagnosed with poly-cystic ovarian syndrome several years ago. She worked with her medical practitioner to balance her hormones, and then began using our products. At last report, she was experiencing hair regrowth and actually adding length to her hair, which had been a challenge before.

Another example of results is my teammate, Jan. Her family members suffer from male and female pattern baldness. The men and women have obvious hair loss. However, since they have been using these products, their scalps are showing less and less all the time. They have had phenomenal results.

Then there is Olivia. Olivia knew her hair was thinning when she started using the products, but had no idea how thin her hair had become on the back of her head. As her hair began to fill in after she started using the products, her friends and family mentioned the back of her head – and that is when she realized just how bad it had been. Hmm, that was me, too. Wow! I guess we humans can convince ourselves of a lot of things that may or may not be accurate.

Everyone will not have the same results because our genetics, the state of our hair follicles (dormant or dead), and medication use vary among each of us. In my opinion, these products provide the best possible choice for thinning hair. They don't contain damaging chemicals and are naturally based. It can take three months or longer for results to be obvious, so be patient.

Hairstyles for Thinning Hair

Have you found the perfect hair style to disguise your thinning hair? Check out these great styles and styling tips along with recommended products to give you the look you want while disguising your thinning hair.

Before

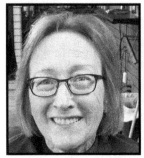 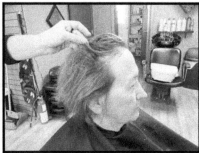

After

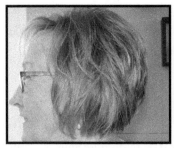 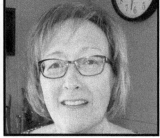

This brave lady has hair loss around the hair line and temple area.

Tips for This Sassy Look:

1. Spritz with Root Lifter on damp hair and apply a small amount of oil on the ends.

2. Blow dry hair all different directions to give more volume.

3. Keep the hair moving at all times while blow drying.

4. Add a few curls with the curling iron and let them fall then spray lightly with refinishing hair spray.

Before

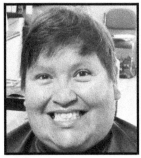 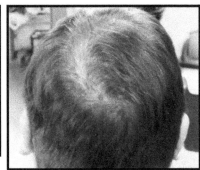

After

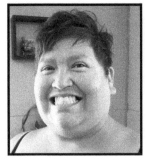 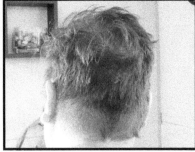

This short and spunky cut is perfect for this brave lady whose hair has filled back in after being able to see her scalp just a few months prior.

Tips for This Spunky Style:

1. Massage in one pump of the Maxie Magnifying Mousse from root to end. Blow dry in a directional manner for a spunkier style.

2. To finish, dip your finger into the Restyle Instant Sculpting Taffy, place it in the palm of your hand and rub your hands together to evenly disperse the product.

3. Add the Taffy to the ends to give it texture and form.

4. Finish with Refinish Control Hair Spray.

Before

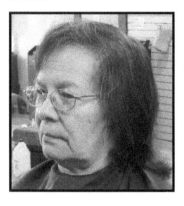
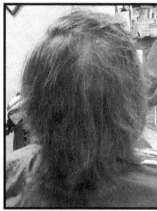

After

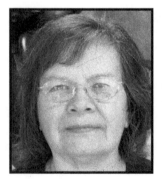
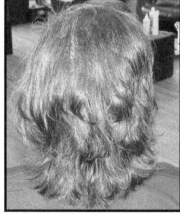

This brave lady has 11 siblings and most are affected by hair loss. She has already had significant regrowth and has some thin areas on top at this time.

Tips to Cover Those Problem Areas:

1. Spritz top of hair with root lifter if starting with dry hair.

2. Wet hair, use the Maxie Magnifying Mousse – one pump distribute from root to ends.

3. Blow dry, keep hair moving in all directions and never stop. It is the best way to get the most volume.

4. Finish with a few curls with the curling iron and spray with Refinish Control Hair Spray.

Before

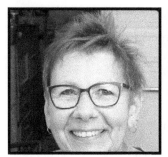
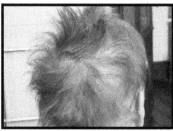

After

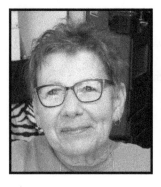
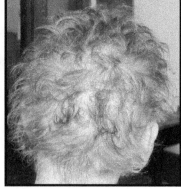

This amazing lady uses humour to talk about her hair loss. She is experiencing some new growth.

Tips for This Fun Style:

1. Use a small amount (less than one pump) of the Moxie Magnifying Mousse, massaging in root to end.

2. Blow dry, keeping the hair moving.

3. Finish with a small amount of the Groom Styling Clay. Place a small amount in the palm of one hand and rub your hands together. Apply to the ends of the hair for texture.

Before

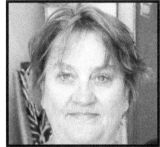

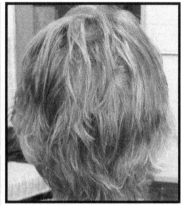

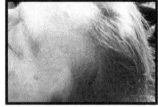

New hair growth
along the hair line.

After

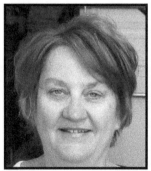

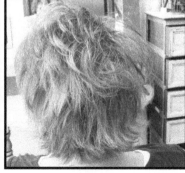

This beautiful lady did not realize how much her hair had regrown until, it was styled by Kelli.

Tips to Get This Much Volume!

1. Instead of a conditioner, use the Junior Gentle Detangler.

2. 4 pumps of the Moxie Magnifying Mousse – massage in root to end.

3. Blow dry.

4. When Dry, spray the Champ Dry Shampoo on the roots for even more volume.

5. Style with the Groom Styling Clay.

Before

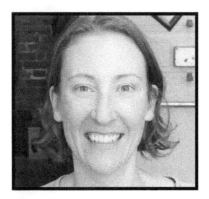

After

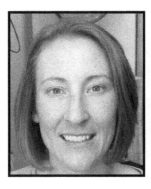
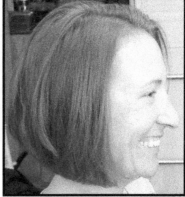

This busy mom has fine, thin hair.

Tips for Getting This Great Volume and Classy Style:

1. Apply a pea-sized amount of the Blow-Out Cream from the roots to the ends.

2. Then, two pumps of the Moxie Magnifying Mousse for volume.

3. Blow dry with a large round brush.

4. Once it is dry, spray the roots with the Champ Dry Shampoo for extra volume.

5. Finish with a light spritz of hair spray.

CHAPTER 5
Real Stories
from Real Women

I n this chapter, I will share stories of real women with you so you can see how some women have treated their hair loss and their results. These are actual people, but I've changed their names to protect their identity. Hair loss can be extremely personal and embarrassing.

Frances

Frances and I had been friends for over ten years before she became my client. She is in her mid-thirties and has

Androgenetic Alopecia as a result of poly-cystic ovarian syndrome (PCOS). She says she started noticing hair loss while she was in high school, was eventually diagnosed with (PCOS), and has been working with her medical practitioner to balance her hormones. I start my initial consult with new clients with an interview process that enables me to learn about the client's hair loss, cause, any previous treatments used, results of previous treatments, and the extensiveness of their hair loss. In addition, the interview gives me the opportunity to connect with my clients and hear where they are emotionally as it relates to their hair loss. Once the interview is complete, I work with my clients to deal with the emotional fall-out and find the best products and solutions for their follicular fall-out. Frances started using Monat's Intensive Repair Treatment System, based on my recommendation, and started seeing hair regrowth after about three months of use. Frances says her hair stylist is not only pleased but surprised at the hair growth she is experiencing. She has new hair growth and her hair length is growing for the first time in several years.

Leona

Leona is the client I mentioned earlier who was almost combative when we first talked. I did not know her before my first consultation with her. She was skeptical because, as she said, she had tried every product and none had worked. She felt that the only alternative, if working with me didn't get her results, would be having hair sewn into her scalp. She has not had to resort to that alternative! The product I recommended for her was the Monat Intense Repair Treatment System.

At first, I was skeptical about working with Leona. I was in Arizona with my husband and daughter visiting our son and his wife for Christmas. I remember it well. We were waiting for the movie *Passengers* to start when she called. I stepped out of the movie theater to talk to her. She almost sounded angry, but now I know that what I heard in her voice was frustration and disappointment in products that promise the moon and don't deliver.

Leona is in her early forties and had diffuse hair loss (all over her head). After just one month, Leona posted before and after pictures. They were of the top of her head before she started using the products and the other one was taken exactly one month later. She was totally thrilled with her results, which were gratifyingly obvious even to a casual observer.

The best part is that I got to meet Leona in person a few months later at an event at a town that was located between each of our respective homes. I reached out to shake her hand when she walked up. She walked right by my hand and gave me the best hug ever!

Heather

I connected with Heather through a post she made on a Facebook page. When I read it, I wanted to know more. Heather is in her mid to late twenties, and had Alopecia Areata. She had actually gotten involved with Monat because of the results she'd had; she wanted to be able to offer the same to others. She says, "I had two months of an exponentially growing bald patch of Alopecia Areata. And that patch was smooth, I'm talking Nair your legs smooth other than about five white hairs. I felt defeated." She shared with me when we were chatting that she had begun withdrawing in general and that her hair loss had strained her relationship with her husband. It was all she thought about, night and day, and so she had basically checked out of her life and relationships as a wife and mom. That is how all-encompassing hair loss can be for women! She began using Monat's Let it Grow System and started seeing results in two weeks. It's also important, in cases like Heather's, that we address the emotional underpinnings, painful thoughts, and limiting beliefs around hair loss, even if that hair loss can be alleviated or even reversed. So much of our self-esteem and our beliefs about our femininity and identity are wrapped up in our hair! Heather did great work, and it only took a few months for her hair to be completely restored.

Jan

Jan is a teammate of mine. In her mid-fifties and one of *12* siblings, she chose to start a Monat business because of all the hair loss in her family. When she joined the team, we had many conversations about the stress her family felt and which product was best for her to use. She started out on one, and then switched. Now, she alternates a couple of the products. She says her six brothers started losing their hair in their twenties. Three of the six women have experienced hair loss; she says some of the women started noticing hair loss while in their thirties. Their father experienced hair loss, though their mother did not.

Jan says she really noticed her hair loss after having a hysterectomy. She had already had thyroid issues and surgery, but her most significant hair loss was after the hysterectomy. One of her sisters had already had some hair loss she thought was caused by a situation where her hair was pulled out. However, once the other sisters began having hair loss, they realized it was not just from that incident.

Jan says her brothers used some of the best-known products on the market with no success. Several of her siblings and Jan use Monat and have had significant hair regrowth. When I first met her, she had more than a widening part. It was more like a part that had an oval area of no hair on top of her head. It is so encouraging to see her hair filling in.

Jan and her daughter are both using Monat and have businesses. Her daughter takes medications for a seizure disorder that causes her hair to fall out. Plus, she knew her family tree had major hair loss in it. It was fun to watch the transformation of Jan's daughter's hair, which started out thin from medication and chemically damaged from hair dyes. Then it was thick and suddenly long! She got a great haircut and her hair was phenomenal. She has such thick black hair now, with a beautiful wave.

Becky

Becky is in her mid-thirties and says she began noticing thinning in the fall of 2016, even though she, like most of us, made excuses for why it was happening. In Becky's case, she decided her hair loss was due to the silk bonnet she'd been sleeping in – maybe the elastic was too tight? – So she replaced it with a scarf. Then, in February, she thought it was looking a little lighter on top. By the end of April, she realized it was definitely lighter on top. This time, she attributed it to the scarf she was wearing and started changing her style.

It was July before she was able to admit that she truly was losing her hair and started Googling everything she could. Becky has learned that one of her medications could cause hair loss. Because that important piece of information was only in the post-marketing material, her medical provider did not realize it could cause hair loss. She worked with her medical provider to stop taking that medication. All of her blood tests have come back normal, and she has an upcoming appointment for scalp biopsies.

Becky has battled depression for years and there many emotional ups and downs with the hair loss. She had a ketamine infusion in May, and she's not sure she could have managed the hair loss with her previous level of depression. The ketamine infusion helped her greatly.

Unfortunately, one of Becky's friends told her that her hair is her defining feature. Needless to say, Becky didn't find that comment helpful. Becky isn't sure when the right time to get a wig is, and hasn't started any type of treatment yet, since she is waiting for the results of her biopsies. She was so scared before the biopsy that she was beside herself.

With clients like Becky who experience extreme stress and anxiety over their hair loss, I recommend they use all the tools in my arsenal to help. Journaling helps release stress and turn around limiting beliefs, and self-care steps help clients relax and focus on other things while we work toward a hair re-growth solution at whatever pace is comfortable for them.

One of the things that was important to Becky's self-esteem was to start wearing make-up, something she hadn't done before, but now does because it helps her feel better about her appearance.

For Becky, showering is so depressing now, seeing the hair in the shower and drain. Every time she sees her hair at the bottom of the tub, it brings up her feelings. Her hair loss is fairly well-disguised at the moment between her hair style and cut, but that doesn't make showering any easier. This is a great reason for powerful mindset work, done right after your shower and especially when dealing with the emotions of hair loss. You need that extra boost to get your day started and have a good attitude to make it through the day.

Flo

I met Flo, a nurse, when she was 58 years old. The great thing for Flo is that as a nurse she knew to be prepared when she went to the doctor. She had researched women's hair loss and knew which tests to request – she asked for iron, thyroid, etc. She says she learned from research that lower iron levels may be considered normal and yet can still affect hair. That's news! Think of it, your iron results are within the normal range so "nothing is wrong with you," and yet there is. The lower end of the "normal" level can still affect your hair.

Flo has used Nioxin and/or Rogaine. She says she could never stay with them long enough to get results because they made her hair look so horrible – she says it was like straw, dry and scraggly. Flo bought a hairpiece hoping it would help, and didn't like it. Now, she keeps her hair cut short so it disguises her hair loss.

Her first doctor ran the tests after she requested them. She chose to take iron and biotin on her own. The second doctor she saw was patient and listened, but acted as though it wasn't a big deal. She says that half the battle is that people take hair loss so after all, it isn't life-threatening!

Flo has had three different occurrences of hair loss, each connected to stress, and each time her hair eventually falls out and grows back over a two-year period. Flo has finally learned to refrain from obsessing over her hair loss. She does say she hates washing her hair – it is just too devastating to see all her hair in the shower and to have to scoop it up to throw it away.

Flo has been proactive and advocated for herself with her medical providers. The next step for clients like Flo is to try switching up products to Monat to keep hair healthy and growing even if they continue so have some hair loss along the way. The idea is to set yourself up to have the best hair health possible to limit hair loss if you are under extreme stress or another physiological affect.

Clients like Flo also deserve the peace of mind that steps in my process to deal with hair loss bring about. Skills to deal with stress, like daily self-care and relaxation techniques, reduce their susceptibility to stress-related hair loss along with regular consultations with me that offer reassurances and answer questions.

CHAPTER 6
What Do You Mean I Am Losing My Hair? Or Denial? I Am Not in Denial!

Those of us with hair loss experience denial in such an insidious way. You think, "I am a woman, I can't be losing my hair!" So you come up with every rationale possible to explain the piles of hair in your shower and those broken pieces covering your bathroom sink where you style your hair every morning. You tell yourself, "It isn't possible that I am losing my hair," yet it consumes you. First we think something like:

- That hair bonnet/ponytail/tight hat/headband I have been wearing is damaging my hair. I'll quit wearing it and see if that helps.

  or...

- It just seems like I am losing more hair than normal. I don't think I really am.

Then, the next tape in the hair loss denial series begins playing over and over in our minds, and includes:

- Am I losing my hair?

- How can it possibly be that I am losing my hair?

- Hair loss is a man's thing, not a woman's thing.

- My hair is so hard to style these days. I wonder what is going on.

One of the scariest parts of denial is its companion, depression. They go hand-in-hand and are like a pair of silent leeches sucking everything out of you as you cut yourself off from relationships and your life. And the person who you think of as your safety net, your medical provider, doesn't realize how depressed you are. They don't even think it is an issue. The denial/depression combo is dangerous because you are in denial and you don't even know yourself how depressed you are.

The good thing that comes out of the denial and depression that come with hair loss is that, for most of us, our resilience and strength eventually win out! I have seen friends and clients experience it, and I have experienced it too. To get to that rallying point, where you're finally ready to take action, though, you need to know what the real reason is behind your denial about your hair loss.

The Real Reason for Denial

So here you are reading this book and nodding your head that yes, you have been in denial about your hair falling out, and really, who needs to know more? That is enough, right? Aw, come on, you already came this far. Let's explore this together.

This next bit is the hardest part of this entire issue, and when you come through it, healing will begin. You think hair loss is the issue or your medical condition that is causing the hair loss. Maybe it's the medication you are taking, or the stress you are under that's the real issue. None of those are it. The biggest issue of all is the damage done to your self-image, your confidence, your self-esteem. That is why you are in denial.

If you admit you are losing your hair, you will come face to face with the confidence you have lost. That is not a comfortable place to be, so you avoid it at all costs. Plus, you are busy enough with everything else you are doing, so why add this insurmountable task of working through your damaged self-esteem?

It really does feel easier, sometimes, to sweep it all under the rug and pretend everything is ok. I want you to know you really are worth the extra effort you will expend to rebuild and reconnect with yourself. I understand, I had lost practically all of my confidence. It was debilitating, and really wasn't who I was.

When you take such a huge hit to your understanding of your inner self, you run the risk of losing "you." You have already pulled away from family, friends, and your normal activities. These are things that define you and give you joy. You have set that aside, and as a result, have set who you are aside.

You begin to let hair loss define you. It starts to become who you are. I know you don't want that, but the hair loss roller coaster picks up so much speed when it goes down that huge decline, it is hard to stop it. You don't know how to stop it even. So you continue to lose more and more of yourself as you pull further and further away from everyone and everything that is important to you. Along the way, you push your emotions deeper and deeper making them almost invisible.

Your hair is a big part of who you are as a person and a woman. It is what you see first thing in the morning in the mirror and what everyone else recognizes about you first. So it is understandable that you are letting your hair loss define who you are as a person.

You are embarrassed and ashamed of the way you look. You think you have done something to deserve thinning hair. Isn't that what our parents said when we did something wrong? "Shame on you!"

How can your hair loss be something you deserve? No one deserves to have their hair fall out and to be embarrassed to be seen in public. You have not done anything to deserve your hair loss.

You need a way to work through the denial, depression, embarrassment and shame. Below I describe a comprehensive 8-step system I developed to help you work through all of these negative emotions. It is my gift to you. You see, I know you can have your life and your joy back all while walking in confidence.

Make a commitment to yourself to follow these steps and start down the road to recovery. It won't be a walk in the park, but you can know that I am walking this path with you.

8 Proven Steps for Dealing with Your Hair Loss

1. **Journal:** Start journaling now even if you aren't sure you are having hair loss or have been dealing with it for years. It is amazing what will come out if you just relax and write freely. It is important to have some music playing in the background that you find relaxing and enjoyable. Choose a notebook that you enjoy seeing and touching. Choose your favorite pen, either for the color of ink, the way it glides across the page, or the way it fits comfortably in your hand. Then, set aside a time each day to journal. Maybe its 15 minutes in the morning before everyone gets up, on your lunch break, or at night after everyone goes to bed. If you don't set aside a time and schedule it, this step likely will not happen and you will lose that opportunity for processing and growth.

2. **Purposeful Relaxation:** I know your day is busy and filled with stress. I find that if I can use a few minutes here and there to de-stress, it makes my entire day much better. Find ways to relax in the nooks and crannies of your day. First, find a quiet place where you can sit and breathe for five minutes. Second, concentrate on your breathing, nothing else (I know bathroom stalls work for this because I have used them for this very thing). Concentrate on your breathing for a full five minutes. Plan some time during breaks, lunch, or before going to be creative. Engaging in a creative outlet, whether creativity means baking a beautiful loaf of bread, singing Karaoke, sewing, painting, or other means of expression, experts say there's a strong connection between creative expression and overall wellbeing. One option that is quick to pull out and put away is to color – yes, color. Adult coloring books have become wildly popular and available at most any store. Find colored pencils or markers you like and keep your supplies in your car or a special drawer at home so if you are feeling stressed and have a minute, you can pull them out and color. I actually color at times on conference calls because I can listen better if my hands are busy. I don't understand it, I just know that it is the case and go with it. Coloring isn't the best option for everyone, for instance, if you are the person that would feel

the need to finish your picture in one sitting and you don't have time for that, choose a different option that fits your time frame.

3. **Choose Safe Effective Products:** Use safe products that have clinically proven ingredients. I and others have used the products I recommend with phenomenal results. While they don't work for everyone, we know exactly how often they work and why they work. And they are safe vs. causing side effects.

4. **Ongoing Support:** One of the most frequent reasons Monat and other hair treatment products don't work is user error including lack of consistent use. You need ongoing support to get the best results possible for you and the best way that can be achieved is through regular, one-on-one support. I have found that I often start a client on one product only to find out that it might not be the best option for them so good and frequent communication is important for the client to continue using the product. In addition, there are plenty of products out there that you can get and use on your own. Not all of them work. I happen to know this one does but the biggest problem is the way it is sold. It is sold with inconsistent support and what I found is my clients were getting mixed results. The ones that are super good at

implementing steps on their own and great at compliance, these are the same people who when their doctor says they need to eat less salt, they eat less salt. I think those people are fantastic, I don't happen to be one of them.

I personally have trouble with compliance and I find that my clients have trouble with compliance too. When I was told to reduce my salt intake, I started craving salt. I know it's one of those mind things. Do you have the same challenges?

I want to be sure you have the best opportunity to get the best results possible. I don't want you to get products and just have them on your shelf collecting dust. My clients have grown their hair back and you can too if you do it correctly but you really need someone reminding you how to do it correctly and troubleshooting any issues along the way. I know after the first 90 days a lot of people develop new habits which is a key to their continued success.

1. **Disguise Your Hair Loss:** Find the best disguising option for you while your hair grows back in. Go back to and look over Chapter Four with the hair loss disguise information in it and choose several methods that will work for you. Journal about them before, during, and after using them to determine if they are the best options for you. Do some

research and find a stylist near you that you are comfortable with and ask for their help. They are masters at hair styling and know just the right products to get you the coverage you need.

2. **Mindset:** This is huge and takes intent on your part. Find an encouraging and positive podcast, music playlist, or audio book and listen to a bit each day. Working on your mindset each and every day is like breathing oxygen. It is a requirement for your survival.

3. **Self-care:** Maybe you think you already do this or maybe you are just going through the motions. Maybe you are not giving yourself any care at all. Whatever the case, let's resolve that right now. What types of self-care really speak to you and make you feel like you are a special person? Is it a massage, a pedicure, a manicure, time at a spiritual retreat by yourself or with friends, or even a hobby? Plan to take time for yourself!

4. **Accountability:** Find an accountability partner that will absolutely hold you accountable and that you can depend on when the journey gets really tough. Otherwise you won't take the steps listed above. It is amazingly difficult for us humans to develop a plan and stick to it without having a

set accountability plan. And, this is extremely difficult work to do on your own. You deserve to have the life you desire with your hair. Do this for you!

These are not skills you will develop overnight. They take practice, perseverance, and the right person to support you in your process. We've all heard that it takes a certain number of days or weeks to instill a new habit. The steps above are no different and take a consistent effort over a long period of time to implement. I believe in you and I know you can do it!

CHAPTER 7
Obstacles and Answers

I n Chapter Five, you read the stories of women who have had different causes for hair loss and have tried a variety of treatments. The stories of these women tell me that some treatments work for a large group of women, some work a little and some don't work at all. I have found that many times, the reason the products haven't worked is because they weren't used correctly and there was no one-on-one support. If you buy a product in a store, there is no one for you to go back to for help using the product in order to get better results. The same is true for products you order online.

There is no one single treatment that works for absolutely everyone, and there is quite a bit of information to sift through. But we can learn from the commonalities among us, the outcome of the treatments tried, and our responses to our experiences. Some are driven to get to the bottom of their hair loss, and others not so much. Let's look at some of the reasons you may choose to avoid taking aggressive steps to resolve your hair loss.

Why Wouldn't You Address Your Hair Loss?

Hair loss is a complicated issue. As a result, there are several reasons why you may not feel up to addressing it. Some of the reasons are information overload; lack of trust due to unscrupulous activity by untrained representatives; misinformation; denial or not accepting that your hair really is thinning; and the lack of validation of the significance of your situation by many in the medical community.

Information overload occurs because there is simply so much information available at your fingertips. In fact, there is so much data out there that it is difficult to digest it all at once. Not only that, some of the information is contradictory! How do you know how to decide what to believe, what to try, and what those crazy-long words that look like a foreign language mean? It is no wonder the information is overwhelming, especially when you are searching night after night with your emotions in the tank. It takes substantial energy and drive just to search the Internet, much less decipher and absorb what you find.

I have observed a fairly strong lack of trust among women with hair loss, and it is well-deserved in many instances. But mistrust can cause you to miss out on innovative solutions, and you never know which solution might work for you. I encourage you to keep an open mind.

Another thing that could prevent you from taking action is misinformation. Company reps are so excited to help you that they may say things that are a little inaccurate, whether purposefully or not. That in turn leads to distrust and the lack of willingness on your part to try a possible solution. Besides, everything else that has promised to regrow hair hasn't worked.

Good ol' denial. It is still not a river in Africa. Denial is refusing to admit the truth or reality of something unpleasant. I talked with several women who said they were in denial at first. This is tough because most of us believe "women don't lose their hair." That is a myth, as you know. This is exactly where I landed. I had worried my entire life that I would be bald because I was the only child in my family that had hair like my dad's. My dad was bald as long as I could remember, only having seen him with hair in pictures.

I don't know if I was in denial because I didn't want to accept it or if I thought it would go away if I buried it deep enough. Denial of hair loss is common in women. After all, it isn't supposed to happen to us.

Remember Becky's story where she kept thinking it was one thing and another that was breaking her hair off instead of realizing she was losing hair? I am certain we women do that type of thing because we have to stay strong for a variety of reasons and it is the only way we can manage at the time. Bury it! That way we can pretend it doesn't exist. Unfortunately, it will eventually become so obvious that we have no option but to deal with it.

Practically every woman with hair loss I've ever talked to has told me that their medical provider had an attitude of, *hey, you still have some hair and you aren't dying, so what's the big deal*? Only one woman reported a different experience. I could not believe how universal a theme that was. It definitely is a huge hurdle in women feeling valued and accepted with their hair loss.

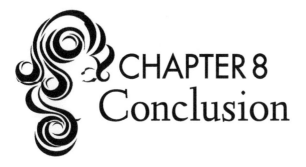

CHAPTER 8
Conclusion

You are not alone, there are over 21,000,000 women in the US alone suffering from hair loss. It is a much larger problem than most people want to admit – me included, until recently. Keep in mind women make up nearly half (40%) of all those suffering from hair loss.

The medical profession could be more sensitive to women with hair loss and that may take a concerted effort by those of us in this community. How else will they know their typical response is traumatizing for women? It is time for women with hair loss to be brave and speak out.

Hair loss is truly a complicated issue with medications, fluctuating hormones, and stress being familiar causes. I have gathered as much information as possible on the causes and treatments for hair loss and included them in this book in words that are clear and easy to understand. The last thing you need to do when you are going through the realization and understanding of hair loss is to try to decipher all those scientific terms. I want to relieve as much stress for you as possible as you travel on this journey.

There are a number of options for disguising your hair loss while waiting for your hair to grow back in. They are described in Chapter Four – choose several that work best for you and use them, embrace them, and make them fun. We need to find ways to have fun during the tough times to get us through.

There are a variety of treatment options. Some "often" work, though we aren't sure why they work, and they are actually derived from a prescription medication for blood pressure. Others have done clinical testing of their ingredients and can tell you how often they work and why. In addition, consider naturally based products over harsh chemicals that can age your skin and affect your blood pressure and heart rate.

I shared stories with you of real women who are still on their hair loss/regrowth journey. These ladies share many of the same traumas and struggles as you. A number of them have come to a place where they know how to manage day to day with less hair, while others are seeing regrowth of their hair they thought they had lost forever.

I also laid out 8 Proven Steps for Dealing with Your Hair Loss. These steps are the most important part of the entire book if you truly want your life back. They are difficult steps, and will require some help along the way. I developed those steps based on my own hair loss journey and coming to terms with it. They are proven actions to move you through the process.

The most important thing to remember is to find the best support you can as you begin your hair loss journey. You need someone who will be there through thick and thin and will work with you through the challenges as well as troubleshoot any issues you have with whatever products you choose. You want someone who has been through the hair loss journey and who can understand where you are coming from and where you want to go.

You deserve to have your hair and your life back, to be able to live again with freedom and spontaneity. Whatever you do, do not let go of that desire. It is up to you to go after your dreams and make them reality. They can be yours.

Acknowledgements

T his book is the result of a journey that started three years ago, my own hair loss journey. I kept it buried for most of these three years. I have had tremendous growth and healing through the amazing naturally based products that worked so well for me, seeing other's results from those products, and the process of writing this book.

This journey would never have happened had Rebecca Elliott not taken a chance and invited me to an event at her salon. My life has been enriched and forever changed as a result. Thank you, Rebecca, for inviting me to your salon that night!

My clients, friends, and others provided the real stories in this book. Without them, it would not have been possible.

I have learned so much about myself and how to release things instead of bury them through this process and as a result of guidance from Melissa Jockheck and coaching and guidance from Angela Lauria. Then, Maggie McReynolds found a way to reach inside and teach me how to give you more of myself, my experience, and my knowledge.

Brittney Canales, my daughter's friend, knows me well and is a breeze to work with. She is flexible and willing to try a variety of shots. Brittney, you always bring out the best of me in pictures.

My family supported me through this process by picking up the slack at home and giving me the freedom to write this book. Thank you Dan and Lora!

My parents taught me to dream and exposed me to a variety of new experiences as a child. Those things along with my passion for helping others fueled me to make the life-long dream of writing a book a reality.

To the Morgan James Publishing team: Special thanks to David Hancock, CEO & Founder for believing in me and my message. To my Author Relations Manager, Bonnie Rauch, thanks for making the process seamless and easy. Many more thanks to everyone else, but especially Jim Howard, Bethany Marshall, and Nickcole Watkins.

Thank You

ongratulations! You are on your way to resolving your hair loss! You have learned how to ride the roller coaster of hair loss and have taken the first step to getting your life back. Take a breath; it is a journey with lots of ups and downs, and I am here to guide you along the way. Please reach out to me to let me know how you are implementing what you have learned as well as your results.

Do you still have questions about what is causing your hair loss? Are you like me and stick to the plan better when you have an accountability system? Has the doctor prescribed a treatment for you like reduced salt in your diet, and you end up craving salt? I get it. That is exactly what happened to me.

The biggest challenge to your success is staying on track and following the steps on your own. If you are like me, you need someone with you along the way.

In order to get you started on your journey the best way possible I have developed a **Free Hair Loss Quiz**. Email me at mjbuckles@icloud.com, with the subject "hair loss quiz". I will get it to you and personally will contact you with your results and an action plan. Let's get you started the right way – and right away.

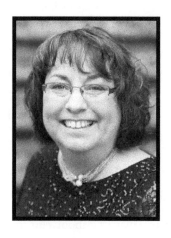

About the Author

Myrna Buckles is passionate about helping others and has completed a 20-year career in the US Public Health Service serving the Indian Health Service and has led short-term mission trips to Nicaragua as well as served in her community. She has a BS in Environmental Science from East Central University in Ada, Oklahoma, and a Master of Science degree in Environmental Health from East Tennessee State University.

Her own experience and that of her clients has given her insight and compassion for women dealing with hair loss. She has guided her clients to the best products for their hair type and hair issue as well as resolving her own hair loss, and, as a result, has built a thriving business. She developed a proven 8-step process to help women deal with their hair loss and regrow their hair.

Website: wigsscarvesandlies.com

Email: myrna@wigsscarvesandlies.com

Facebook: https://www.facebook.com/myrna.buckles

LinkedIn: https://www.linkedin.com/in/myrna-buckles

Appendix

Drug Induced
Hair Loss

Many commonly prescribed prescription drugs can cause temporary hair loss, trigger the onset of male and female pattern baldness, and even cause permanent hair loss. Note that the drugs listed here do not include those used in chemotherapy and radiation for cancer treatment.

Your doctor may not mention hair loss as a side effect of some drugs, so don't forget to do your own research and read the drug manufacturer's complete warnings. Your pharmacist can provide you with this information even before you fill a prescription.

Many pill and medication guidebooks (sold in bookstores and pharmacies) are also excellent sources of complete information about prescription drugs. If your doctor prescribes any of the following drugs, ask if one that does not have hair loss as a possible side effect can be substituted.

The drugs are listed by category, according to the conditions they treat, then by brand name first, followed by the drug's generic name in parentheses. In some categories, individual drugs are not listed. For these conditions, you will want to discuss the possibility of hair loss as a side effect of using any of the drugs that treat that particular condition, since many do contribute to hair loss.

Acne	All drugs derived from vitamin A as treatments for acne or other conditions, including: • Accutane (isotretinoin)
Blood	Anticoagulants (bloodthinners), including: • Panwarfin (warfarinsodium) • Sofarin (warfarinsodium) • Coumadin (warfarinsodium) • Heparininjections
Cholesterol	Cholesterol-loweringdrugs, including: • Atronid-S (clofibrate) • Lopid (gemfibrozil)

Convulsions/ Epilepsy	• Anticonvulsants, including: • Tridone (trimethadione)
Depression	• Antidepressiondrugs, including: • Prozac (fluoxetinehydrochloride) • Zoloft (sertralinehydrochloride) • Paxil (paroxetine) • Anafranil (clomipramine) • Janimine (imipramine) • Tofranil (imipramine) • Tofranil PM (imipramine) • Adapin (doxepin) • Sinequan (doxepin) • Surmontil (trimipramine) • Pamelor (nortriptyline) • Ventyl (nortriptyline) • Elavin (amitriptyline) • Endep (amitriptyline) • Norpramin (desipramine) • Pertofrane (desipramine) • Vivactil (protriptylinehydrochloride) • Asendin (amoxapine) • Haldol (haloperidol)
Diet	• Amphetamines
Fungus	• Antifungals
Glaucoma	The beta-blocker drugs, including: • TimopticEyeDrops (timolol) • TimopticOcudose (timolol) • Timoptic XC (timolol)
Gout	• Lopurin (allopurinol) • Zyloprim (allopurinol)

Heart	• Tenormin (atenolol) • Lopressor (metoprolol) • Corgard (nadolol) • Inderal and Inderal LA (propanolol) • Blocadren (timolol)
High Blood Pressure	See Above list of beta blockers under "Heart"
Hormonal Conditions	All hormone-containing drugs and drugs prescribed for hormone-related, reproductive, male-specific, and female-specific conditions and situations have the potential to cause hair loss, including: • Birth Control Pills • Hormone-replacement therapy (HRT) for women (estrogen or progesterone) • Male androgenic hormones and all forms of testosterone • Anabolicsteriods • Prednisone and othersteroids
Parkinson's Disease	• Levadopa / L-dopa (dopar, larodopa)
Thyroid Disorders	• Many of the drugs used to treat the thyroid
Ulcer	Many of the drugs used to treat indigestion, stomach difficulties, and ulcers, including over-the-counter dosages and prescription dosages. • Tagamet (cimetidine) • Zantac (ranitidine) • Pepcid (famotidine)

Inflammation	Many anti-inflammatory drugs, including those prescribed for localized pain, swelling and injury.
	• Arthritisdrugs
	• Nonsteroidal Anti-Inflammatory Drugs including:
	• Naprosyn (naproxen)
	• Anaprox (naproxen)
	• Anaprox DS (naproxen)
	• Indocin (indomethacin)
	• Indocin SR (indomethacin)
	• Clinoril (sulindac)
	An anti-inflammatory that is also used as a chemotherapy drug:
	• Methotrexate (MTX)
	• Rheumatex (methotrexate)
	• Folex (methotrexate)

Reviewed by Paul J. McAndrews, MD

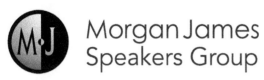

Morgan James
Speakers Group

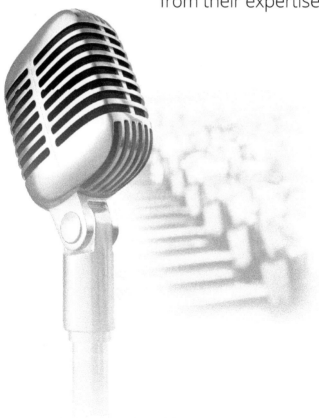

www.TheMorganJamesSpeakersGroup.com

We connect Morgan James published
authors with live and online events
and audiences who will benefit
from their expertise.

CPSIA information can be obtained
at www.ICGtesting.com
Printed in the USA
BVHW080358081218
535094BV00002B/12/P